low energy help for men

A Guide to Boosting Your Energy and Living Your Best Life

hunter hazelton

contents

introduction

Low energy is a problem that affects many men, yet it is often overlooked or dismissed as a natural part of getting older. But the truth is that low energy can have a significant impact on men's health and wellbeing, and can negatively affect their daily lives.

Energy is the fuel that powers our bodies and minds. Without it, we struggle to perform even the simplest of tasks, and our quality of life suffers. For men, energy is especially important, as they are often expected to be the breadwinners and providers for their families. Whether at work, at home, or in their personal lives, men need energy to be able to meet the demands placed upon them.

Unfortunately, many men experience low energy at some point in their lives. This can be caused by a number of factors, including poor nutrition, lack of exercise, inadequate sleep, high stress levels, and hormonal imbalances. Understanding the root causes of low energy is the first step in addressing the problem and finding effective solutions.

The purpose of this book is to provide men with a comprehensive guide to boosting their energy levels and living their best lives. We will explore the common causes of low energy in men and provide practical tips and strategies for overcoming them. Our goal is to help men regain their energy and vitality, so that they can thrive in all areas of their lives.

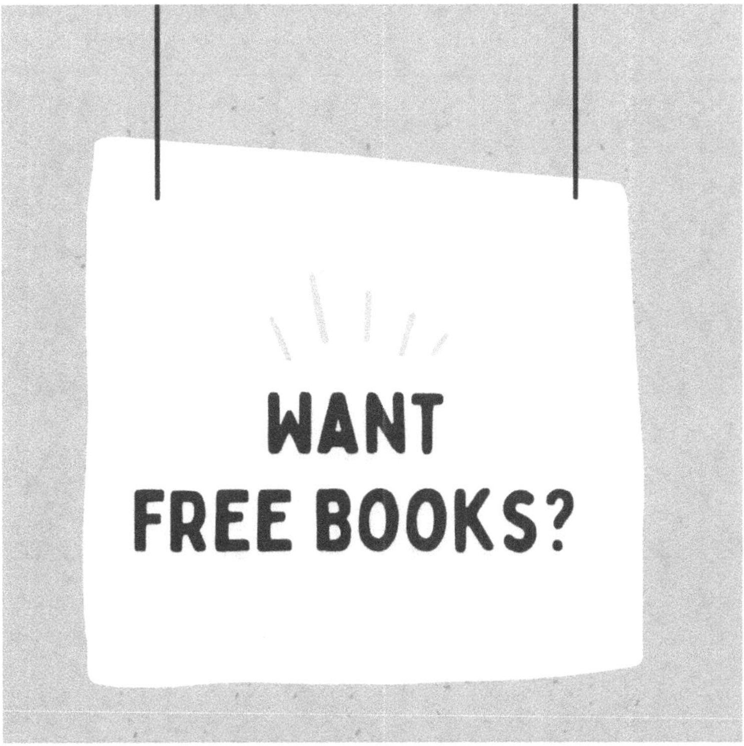

WANT
FREE BOOKS?
FREEBOOKDAILY.COM

SKY HIGH ENERGY BILL?

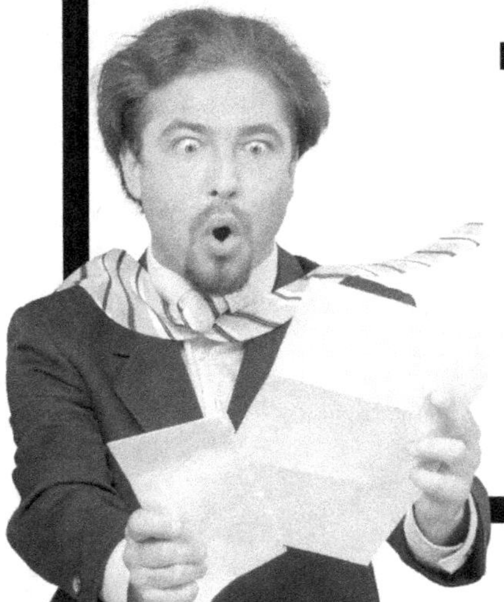

understanding low energy

. . .

"A real man never stops trying to show his woman how much she means to him, even after he's got her."

Anonymous

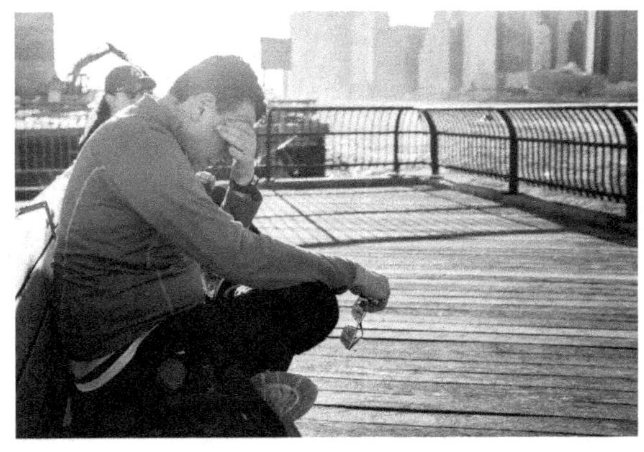

What is Low Energy and Why it Matters

LOW ENERGY. It's like a flat tire on a rainy day. You're stuck, going nowhere fast, and it just feels like the universe is conspiring against you. But here's the thing, fellas. Low energy matters. It's not just about feeling tired all the time. It's about how it affects every aspect of your life.

THINK OF IT LIKE A BIG, beautiful engine. You're the driver, and that engine is your body and mind. When that engine is running smoothly, you can go anywhere you want. But when it's sputtering and struggling to keep up, well, it's not exactly a joyride.

LOW ENERGY CAN IMPACT your work life. You know that feeling when you're sitting at your desk, staring at the screen, and it feels like your brain is made of molasses? Yeah, that's low energy. It can make it harder to focus, harder to be productive, and harder to get things done.

. . .

BUT IT'S NOT JUST work. Low energy can impact your relationships, too. When you're feeling drained and exhausted, it's harder to be present for your loved ones. You might snap at them, or withdraw, or just not have the energy to do the things you used to enjoy together.

AND LET'S not forget about your health. When your energy is low, it can be harder to motivate yourself to exercise, eat well, and take care of your body. And that can lead to a whole host of problems down the road.

BUT HERE'S the good news, guys. You don't have to accept low energy as a fact of life. There are things you can do to boost your energy levels and get that engine revving again.

The Importance of Energy for Men's Health and Wellbeing

ENERGY IS a fundamental aspect of a man's health and wellbeing. It's the fuel that powers our bodies and minds, allowing us to tackle life's challenges with vigor and determination. But when our energy levels are low, it can feel like we're slogging through quicksand, struggling to keep up with the demands of our daily lives.

THE TRUTH IS, low energy isn't just a minor inconvenience. It can have a significant impact on our physical and mental health, as well as our overall quality of life. When we're low on energy, we're more susceptible to illness, injury, and chronic health conditions. We may find it harder to concentrate, make decisions, and engage with the world around us. And we may experience feelings of depression, anxiety, and other mental health issues.

THE IMPORTANCE of energy for men's health and wellbeing cannot be overstated. It's not just about feeling good in the moment. It's about investing in our long-term health and happiness. When we prioritize our energy levels, we're taking a proactive approach to our health, setting ourselves up for success and vitality in the years to come.

So, what exactly is energy, and how does it impact our health? At its most basic level, energy is the ability to do work. It's what allows us to move, think, and feel. Energy comes from the food we eat, the air we breathe, and the way we move our bodies. When we're low on energy, it can manifest in a variety of ways, including fatigue, weakness, and lethargy.

WHEN WE HAVE high energy levels, we're better equipped to handle the demands of our daily lives. We're more productive at work, more engaged with our families, and more likely to pursue our passions and hobbies. We have greater mental clarity and focus, allowing us to make better decisions and solve problems more effectively. And we're more resilient in the face of stress and adversity, able to bounce back from setbacks and keep moving forward.

So, how can we boost our energy levels and take control of our health and wellbeing? There are a variety of strategies we can use, ranging from basic lifestyle changes to more targeted interventions. Some of the most effective methods for boosting energy levels include:

- Eating a balanced, nutrient-dense diet that provides the fuel our bodies need to function optimally
- Engaging in regular exercise that supports our physical and mental health
- Prioritizing sleep and rest, allowing our bodies to recharge and recover

- Managing stress effectively, reducing the wear and tear on our bodies and minds
- Addressing any underlying health issues or imbalances that may be contributing to low energy levels

By implementing these strategies and making energy a priority in our lives, we can experience the many benefits that come with high energy levels. We'll feel better physically, mentally, and emotionally, allowing us to live our lives to the fullest and achieve our goals and aspirations.

This book will dive into the specifics to help you regain the energy levels you felt as a kid while helping you understand how specific actions fit into the overall framework of a more energetic lifestyle. Better energy doesn't always happen overnight, but believe it or not, there are simple actions you can incorporate into today, that will transform your tomorrow!

The Common Causes of Low Energy in Men

Low energy is a common problem that affects many men, and there are a variety of factors that can contribute to this issue. Understanding the root causes of low energy is essential for developing effective strategies to address it and regain our vitality and vigor. Here are some of the most common causes of low energy in men:

- Poor Nutrition: What we eat plays a significant role in our energy levels. Consuming a diet that is high in processed and sugary foods, lacking in essential vitamins and minerals, and low in protein and healthy fats can leave us feeling tired and sluggish.
- Lack of Exercise: Exercise is essential for maintaining our physical and mental health, and it's also critical for boosting our energy levels. Regular exercise increases blood flow, improves cardiovascular health, and enhances overall energy levels.
- Inadequate Sleep: Sleep is essential for allowing our bodies to recover and recharge. When we don't get enough quality sleep, our bodies and minds suffer, leading to fatigue and low energy levels.
- High Stress Levels: Chronic stress can take a significant toll on our bodies and minds, leading to exhaustion and burnout. Finding effective ways to manage stress is critical for maintaining high energy levels.

- Hormonal Imbalances: Hormonal imbalances can contribute to low energy levels in men. Low testosterone, for example, can lead to fatigue, decreased muscle mass, and other symptoms that impact our energy levels.
- Dehydration: Even mild dehydration can lead to fatigue and low energy levels. Ensuring that we're adequately hydrated throughout the day is critical for maintaining our energy levels.
- Medications: Certain medications, including those used to treat high blood pressure, depression, and anxiety, can contribute to low energy levels as a side effect.
- Chronic Health Conditions: Chronic health conditions such as diabetes, heart disease, and autoimmune disorders can impact our energy levels and lead to fatigue.

UNDERSTANDING these common causes of low energy in men is the first step in developing effective strategies to address them. By making lifestyle changes, seeking medical treatment when necessary, and prioritizing our energy levels, we can take control of our health and well-being and regain our vitality and vigor.

How Low Energy Can Affect Your Daily Life

Low energy can have a significant impact on our daily lives, affecting everything from our work performance to our relationships and overall quality of life. Here are some of the ways that low energy can impact us on a day-to-day basis:

- Decreased Productivity: Low energy can make it challenging to concentrate and stay focused, leading to decreased productivity at work or school.
- Lack of Motivation: When we're low on energy, it can be difficult to find the motivation to do even the simplest tasks, such as household chores or exercise.
- Mood Swings: Low energy levels can lead to irritability, mood swings, and a general feeling of malaise, making it harder to interact with others in a positive and constructive way.
- Relationship Strain: Low energy can impact our relationships with others, making it harder to engage with our loved ones and leading to feelings of isolation and disconnection.

- Reduced Physical Performance: Low energy can impact our physical performance, making it harder to engage in physical activity, sports, and other activities that require stamina and endurance.
- Decreased Cognitive Function: Low energy levels can lead to brain fog, memory problems, and other cognitive issues that impact our ability to think clearly and make decisions effectively.
- Weight Gain: Low energy levels can lead to overeating, weight gain, and other health issues that impact our overall quality of life.
- Lack of Sleep: Low energy levels can impact our ability to get a good night's sleep, leading to a vicious cycle of fatigue and sleep deprivation.
- Mental Health Issues: Chronic low energy levels can lead to depression, anxiety, and other mental health issues that impact our overall wellbeing.

It's clear that low energy can have a significant impact on our daily lives, affecting everything from our work performance to our relationships and overall quality of life. By taking steps to address the root causes of low energy, we can regain our vitality and vigor, and live our lives to the fullest.

Symptoms of Low Energy

LOW ENERGY IS a common problem that many people experience in their daily lives. It can be caused by a variety of factors, including poor nutrition, lack of exercise, stress, and medical conditions. Regardless of the cause, low energy can significantly impact our daily lives, affecting everything from our productivity at work to our ability to engage with loved ones and participate in activities that we enjoy.

ONE OF THE most common ways that low energy can manifest is through physical symptoms. People with low energy levels may feel physically fatigued, as though they're carrying around a weight that makes it difficult to move and perform daily tasks. They may also experience muscle aches and pains, headaches, and dizziness, which can make it difficult to focus and concentrate on tasks.

IN ADDITION TO PHYSICAL SYMPTOMS, low energy can also impact our mood and emotional wellbeing. People with low energy levels may feel irritable, anxious, or depressed, making it difficult to interact with others in a positive way. They may also feel unmotivated and lack the drive to accomplish tasks or pursue hobbies and interests that they once enjoyed.

LOW ENERGY CAN ALSO IMPACT our ability to be productive at work or school. People with low energy levels may find it difficult to concentrate and stay focused, leading to decreased productivity and lower-quality work. They may also struggle to complete tasks that require physical effort, such as lifting heavy objects or standing for long periods of time.

SOCIALLY, low energy can also impact our ability to engage with loved ones and participate in activities that we enjoy. People with low energy levels may feel too tired or drained to engage in social activities, preferring to stay home and rest instead. This can lead to feelings of isolation and loneliness, which can further impact our emotional wellbeing.

LOW ENERGY CAN ALSO IMPACT our physical health over time. People with low energy levels may be less likely to engage in physical activity, leading to weight gain and other health problems. They may also be more susceptible to illness and injury, as their bodies are less able to fight off infections and heal from injuries.

MOST IMPORTANTLY, low energy can mean that our spouse or children do not receive the attention and focus they deserve. While we might remember the good old days, those closest to us may only know one version of us, **The Tired Version**. For me nothing is worse then when I think my family is getting the short end of the stick because I have given what little energy I have to a job that might replace me and a boss who could fire me tomorrow without a second thought. Our families and friends care about us on a deeper level and we are more than just a number to the ones who count on us for everything. My hope is that this book helps inspire you to take the necessary action to regain your life, and teaches you the practical tools to make that a reality!

the science of energy

. . .

"A real man loves his wife, and places his family
as the most important thing in life. Nothing has
brought me more peace and content in life than
simply being a good husband and father."

Frank Abagnale

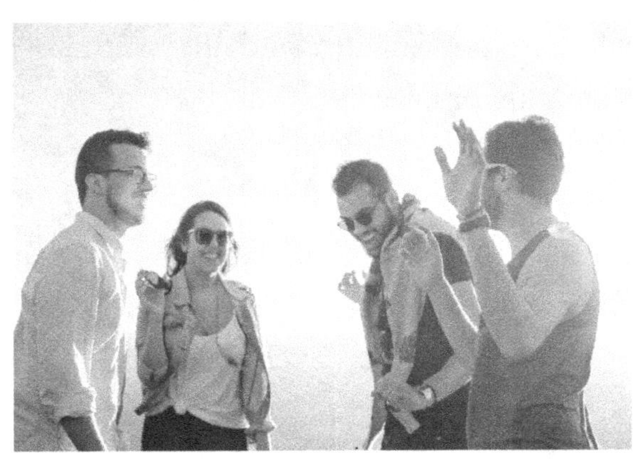

The Science Behind Energy Production

ENERGY IS essential for all living organisms, including humans. Our bodies require energy to function properly, from powering our muscles to maintaining our internal organs. The process of energy production is complex and involves numerous systems and processes within our bodies. Here's a closer look at the science behind energy production.

ENERGY IS PRODUCED within our cells through a process called cellular respiration. This process involves breaking down glucose (a type of sugar) into a molecule called adenosine triphosphate (ATP), which is the primary energy currency of our cells. ATP provides the energy needed for all of our cellular processes, including muscle contraction, nerve signaling, and the synthesis of new proteins and other molecules.

CELLULAR RESPIRATION IS a multi-step process that occurs in several stages, including glycolysis, the Krebs cycle, and the electron transport chain. During glycolysis, glucose is broken down into pyruvate, which is then converted into acetyl-CoA and enters the Krebs cycle. The Krebs cycle produces a small amount of ATP directly and also generates electron carriers that are used in the electron transport chain to produce additional ATP.

THE ELECTRON TRANSPORT chain is the final stage of cellular respiration and is where the majority of ATP is produced. During this process, electrons are passed along a series of enzymes and protein complexes, generating a gradient of protons (positively charged particles) across the inner membrane of mitochondria. This proton gradient is then used to power the synthesis of ATP through an enzyme called ATP synthase.

WHILE CELLULAR RESPIRATION is the primary way that our bodies produce energy, there are other systems and processes that also play a role. For example, the breakdown of fats and proteins can also generate ATP through a process called beta-oxidation. Additionally, the metabolism of carbohydrates and other nutrients in our diets provides the building blocks needed for energy production.

.   .   .

THE PROCESS of energy production is tightly regulated by several systems within our bodies. One of the most important is the endocrine system, which produces hormones that regulate metabolism and energy balance. Hormones like insulin, glucagon, and cortisol help to maintain blood glucose levels and ensure that our cells have the nutrients they need for energy production.

OTHER SYSTEMS that play a role in energy production include the circulatory system, which transports oxygen and nutrients to our cells, and the nervous system, which helps to regulate the activity of our muscles and organs.

IT'S easy to see that energy production is a complex process that involves numerous systems and processes within our bodies. Cellular respiration is the primary way that our cells generate ATP, the energy currency that powers all of our cellular processes. Other systems, such as the endocrine, circulatory, and nervous systems, also play important roles in energy production and regulation. Understanding the science behind energy production can help us make informed decisions about our diet, exercise habits, and overall health and wellbeing.

Types of Energy

THERE ARE several types of energy that are essential for our bodies to function properly. Here are some of the most important types of energy that help our bodies function each and everyday:

- Chemical Energy: Chemical energy is the energy stored in the bonds between molecules and is essential for many of the body's metabolic processes. Our bodies use chemical energy from food to fuel the creation of ATP, the primary energy currency of our cells.
- Electrical Energy: Electrical energy is essential for the proper functioning of our nervous system, which uses electrical impulses to transmit information between cells. Our brains and muscles also rely on electrical energy to function properly.
- Thermal Energy: Our bodies need thermal energy to maintain a constant internal temperature and to regulate many of our bodily processes. When we are too cold or too hot, our bodies work to regulate our internal temperature through processes like shivering, sweating, and vasodilation.
- Radiant Energy: Radiant energy, specifically in the form of sunlight, is essential for the production of vitamin D in our bodies.

Vitamin D is important for bone health and
helps to regulate our immune system.

- Kinetic Energy: Our bodies rely on kinetic
  energy to move and perform physical tasks.
  This includes everything from running and
  jumping to breathing and digesting food.
- Potential Energy: Potential energy is stored
  energy that can be converted into other forms
  of energy. For example, the potential energy
  stored in the chemical bonds of food can be
  converted into kinetic energy for movement
  and activity.

IN CONCLUSION, there are several types of energy that are
essential for our bodies to function properly. From chemical
energy that powers our metabolism to electrical
energy that allows our nerves and muscles to communicate, each type of energy plays an important role in
keeping our bodies healthy and functioning properly.

Measuring Energy Levels

WHEN WE WERE YOUNGER, we might not have thought
much about our energy levels. We ran around and played

without a second thought, fueled by the boundless energy of youth. But as we get older, we start to become more aware of our energy levels and how they impact our daily lives. Measuring our energy levels becomes more important, just like measuring the amount of fuel in a car before a long road trip.

Just like a car needs fuel to run, our bodies need energy to function properly. When our energy levels are low, we may feel sluggish, unmotivated, and unable to perform even the simplest tasks. It's like running on empty, trying to drive a car without any gas in the tank.

But just like we can monitor the fuel gauge in a car, we can measure our energy levels to ensure that we have enough energy to get through the day. This might mean taking note of how we feel throughout the day, paying attention to the foods we eat, and making sure to get enough sleep and exercise. It's like checking the oil and tire pressure in a car before a long trip to make sure that everything is running smoothly.

Think of measuring energy levels like a battery indicator on a phone or laptop. Just like a battery needs to be charged to function properly, our bodies need to be fueled with energy to function at our best. We can monitor our energy levels throughout the day, just like we can monitor the battery level on our devices, and take steps to recharge when our energy levels start to dip. The secret is learning the specific indications our bodies gives us to help us measure that reading!

nutrition and energy

. . .

"Being male is a matter of birth. Being a man is a matter of age. But being a gentleman is a matter of choice."

Vin Diesel

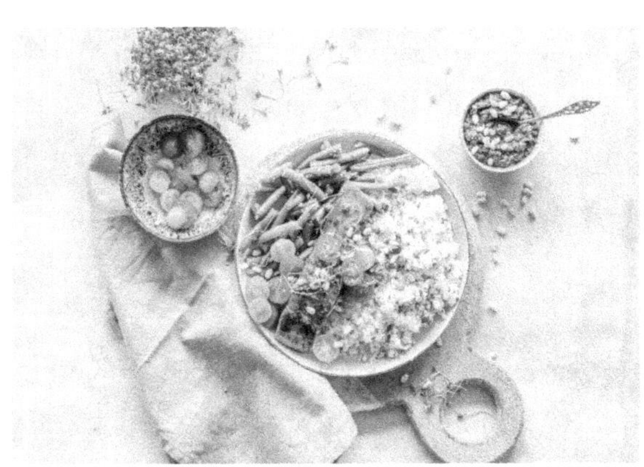

The Role of Nutrition in Energy Production

NUTRITION PLAYS a critical role in energy production in our bodies. The foods we eat provide the building blocks and nutrients needed for our cells to generate energy through cellular respiration. Without adequate nutrition, our bodies cannot produce the energy needed for daily activities, which can lead to feelings of fatigue and lethargy.

ONE OF THE key nutrients involved in energy production is carbohydrates. Carbohydrates are broken down into glucose, which is used as the primary fuel for cellular respiration. Complex carbohydrates, such as whole grains and vegetables, provide a sustained source of energy, while simple carbohydrates, such as sugar and refined flour, can provide a quick boost of energy but are often followed by a crash.

PROTEIN IS another important nutrient involved in energy production. Amino acids, the building blocks of protein, can be broken down and converted into glucose through a process called gluconeogenesis. Protein is also involved in the synthesis of enzymes and other molecules involved in cellular respiration.

Fats are also an important source of energy for our bodies. Fats are broken down into fatty acids and glycerol, which can be converted into ATP through a process called beta-oxidation. Fats provide a long-lasting source of energy and are particularly important during endurance exercise.

In addition to macronutrients like carbohydrates, protein, and fat, micronutrients like vitamins and minerals are also important for energy production. B vitamins, for example, are involved in the breakdown of carbohydrates and the synthesis of ATP, while minerals like iron and magnesium are involved in oxygen transport and muscle function.

A balanced and varied diet is essential for optimal energy production in our bodies. Eating a diet rich in whole grains, vegetables, fruits, lean protein, and healthy fats can provide the nutrients needed for energy production and help to prevent feelings of fatigue and lethargy. On the other hand, a diet high in processed foods and refined carbohydrates can lead to spikes and crashes in energy levels and may contribute to feelings of fatigue and low energy.

Foods that Boost and Drain Energy

THE FOODS we eat play a significant role in our energy levels. Some foods can provide a quick boost of energy, while others can leave us feeling sluggish and drained. By making smart choices about the foods we eat, we can ensure that we have the energy we need to power through our day.

FOODS THAT BOOST energy tend to be high in complex carbohydrates, protein, and fiber. These nutrients provide sustained energy and can help to prevent spikes and crashes in energy levels. Examples of foods that boost energy include whole grains, fruits and vegetables, nuts and seeds, lean protein sources like chicken and fish, and healthy fats like avocado and olive oil.

ON THE OTHER HAND, foods that drain energy tend to be high in sugar, refined carbohydrates, and unhealthy fats. These foods can provide a quick burst of energy, but often leave us feeling tired and lethargic. Examples of foods that drain energy include sugary snacks and beverages, processed foods like chips and crackers, fried foods, and fast food.

SURPRISINGLY, some foods can do either, depending on the amount and timing of consumption. For example, coffee and tea can provide a quick boost of energy, but too much caffeine can lead to jitters and crashes. Similarly, while alcohol can initially provide a feeling of relaxation and euphoria, it can also lead to fatigue and dehydration.

Foods That Boost Energy

- Oatmeal
- Quinoa
- Bananas
- Blueberries
- Sweet potatoes
- Salmon
- Almonds
- Greek yogurt
- Eggs
- Spinach
- Broccoli

- Black beans
- Edamame
- Lentils
- Green tea
- Dark chocolate
- Chia seeds
- Pumpkin seeds
- Avocado
- Olive oil

Foods That Drain Energy

- Candy
- Soda
- Energy drinks - *After a short-lived energy spike
- Fast food
- Processed meats
- White bread
- French fries
- Potato chips
- Donuts
- Cake
- Ice cream
- Bacon

- Pizza
- Fried chicken
- Alcohol
- Sugary cereal
- White rice
- Margarine
- Artificial sweeteners
- High-fructose corn syrup

THE FOODS we eat can have a significant impact on our energy levels. By making smart choices and opting for foods that provide sustained energy and avoiding those that lead to crashes, we can ensure that we have the energy we need to power through our day. Surprisingly, some foods can do either, depending on the amount and timing of consumption, so it's important to pay attention to how our bodies react to different foods.

Meal Planning for Sustained Energy

MEAL PLANNING IS an important part of maintaining sustained energy levels throughout the day. By choosing the right combination of foods and nutrients, we can ensure that our bodies have the energy they need to power through our day.

ONE MEAL PLANNING strategy is to focus on nutrient-dense foods that provide sustained energy. This might include whole grains, fruits and vegetables, lean protein sources, and healthy fats. Meals should be balanced and include a mix of macronutrients like carbohydrates, protein, and fat. Snacks can also be an important part of meal planning, providing an energy boost between meals.

ANOTHER MEAL PLANNING strategy is to plan ahead for busy days or times when healthy eating might be more challenging. This might involve preparing meals and snacks in advance, packing healthy snacks to take on the go, or choosing healthy options when eating out.

WHEN IT COMES to combining multiple energy-producing foods into a super meal, there are a few key strategies to keep in mind. First, aim for a mix of carbohydrates, protein, and healthy fats in each meal. This might mean choosing a whole grain, like quinoa or brown rice, as a base and adding a protein source like chicken or tofu, along with healthy fats like avocado or nuts.

· · ·

ANOTHER STRATEGY IS to incorporate foods that are high in specific nutrients that are important for energy production. For example, iron is essential for oxygen transport in the body and can be found in foods like spinach, lentils, and beef. Magnesium is also important for energy production and can be found in foods like almonds, avocados, and dark chocolate. Here's an example of a super meal that combines multiple energy-producing foods:

- Grilled chicken breast seasoned with herbs and spices
- Quinoa cooked with chicken broth and mixed with roasted vegetables like bell peppers, onions, and zucchini
- A side of roasted sweet potato wedges seasoned with cinnamon and paprika
- A small serving of dark chocolate or fresh fruit for dessert

THIS MEAL PROVIDES a mix of carbohydrates, protein, and healthy fats, along with important nutrients like iron and magnesium. By combining multiple energy-producing foods into a single meal, we can ensure that our bodies have the sustained energy they need to power through our day.

. . .

IN CONCLUSION, meal planning is an important part of maintaining sustained energy levels throughout the day. By choosing the right combination of foods and nutrients and incorporating multiple energy-producing foods into super meals, we can ensure that our bodies have the energy they need to thrive. Whether we're planning meals for busy weekdays or special occasions, there are many strategies we can use to support our energy levels and overall health.

exercise and energy

. . .

"A man's true character comes out when he's drunk."

Charlie Chaplin

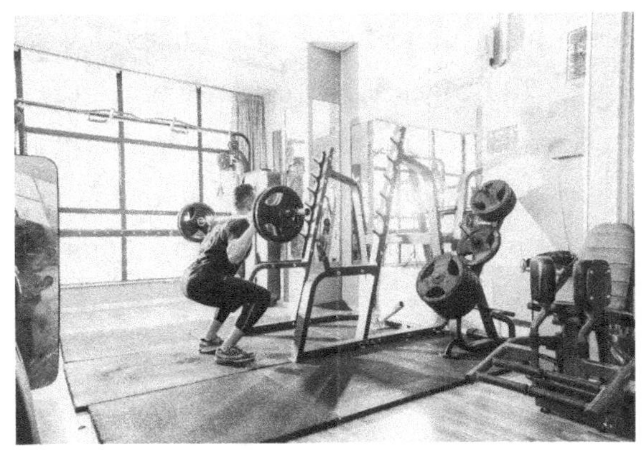

Exercise and Energy Production

EXERCISE PLAYS a critical role in energy production in our bodies. Regular physical activity helps to improve the efficiency of our cardiovascular and respiratory systems, which in turn allows our bodies to produce energy more efficiently. Exercise also stimulates the production of mitochondria, the powerhouses of our cells, which are responsible for producing ATP, the primary energy currency of our cells.

WHEN WE EXERCISE, our bodies use a mix of carbohydrates and fats for fuel. During low-intensity exercise, our bodies primarily rely on fat stores for energy, while during high-intensity exercise, our bodies rely more heavily on carbohydrates. By regularly engaging in physical activity, we can improve our bodies' ability to use both carbohydrates and fats for fuel, allowing us to exercise for longer periods of time and with greater intensity.

REGULAR EXERCISE also helps to improve insulin sensitivity, which is essential for proper glucose metabolism and energy production. This can help to prevent insulin resistance, a condition in which the body becomes less responsive to insulin, leading to high blood sugar levels and a decrease in energy production.

IN ADDITION to improving energy production, exercise can also help to reduce feelings of fatigue and improve overall mood. Regular physical activity stimulates the release of endorphins, neurotransmitters that promote feelings of wellbeing and happiness. Exercise also helps to reduce stress, which can contribute to feelings of fatigue and low energy.

OVERALL, regular exercise is essential for optimal energy production and overall health. By engaging in physical activity on a regular basis, we can improve our bodies' ability to produce energy efficiently, reduce feelings of fatigue, and improve overall mood and wellbeing. Whether we're engaging in low-intensity activities like walking or high-intensity activities like running, regular exercise is an important part of maintaining our energy levels and overall health.

Best Exercises for Boosting Energy

While any type of physical activity can help to boost energy levels, some exercises are particularly effective at improving energy production and reducing feelings of fatigue. Here are some of the best exercises for boosting energy:

- Cardiovascular Exercise: Any type of cardiovascular exercise, such as running, cycling, or swimming, can help to improve energy levels. Cardiovascular exercise improves cardiovascular and respiratory function, which allows our bodies to produce energy more efficiently.
- High-Intensity Interval Training (HIIT): HIIT involves short bursts of high-intensity exercise followed by periods of rest or lower intensity exercise. HIIT has been shown to improve energy production and reduce fatigue, making it a great choice for boosting energy levels.
- Yoga: Yoga combines physical movement with mindfulness and relaxation techniques, making it a great choice for reducing stress and improving energy levels. Yoga also helps to improve flexibility, balance, and strength.
- Resistance Training: Resistance training, such as weight lifting or bodyweight exercises, helps to improve muscular strength and endurance,

which can improve overall energy levels. Resistance training also helps to improve insulin sensitivity, which is important for proper glucose metabolism and energy production.

- Walking: While it may seem simple, walking is a great way to boost energy levels. Walking improves cardiovascular and respiratory function and can help to reduce stress, making it a great choice for improving energy levels.

WHEN IT COMES to boosting energy levels through exercise, it's important to find activities that you enjoy and that fit into your lifestyle. Whether you're engaging in high-intensity exercise or low-impact activities like walking or yoga, regular physical activity is essential for maintaining optimal energy levels and overall health.

HERE ARE 25 weight training exercises broken down by body part to help increase energy:

CHEST:

- Bench press
- Push-ups

- Chest flys
- Cable crossovers
- Dumbbell pullovers

BACK:

- Pull-ups
- Lat pulldowns
- Seated cable rows
- T-bar rows
- Deadlifts

SHOULDERS:

- Military press
- Arnold press
- Lateral raises
- Rear delt flys
- Upright rows

ARMS:

- Bicep curls

- Hammer curls
- Tricep extensions
- Skull crushers
- Cable curls

Legs:

- Squats
- Lunges
- Leg press
- Leg curls
- Calf raises

These exercises target major muscle groups in the body, promoting muscle growth and improved energy levels. By incorporating weight training exercises into your workout routine, you can improve overall strength and endurance, which can lead to improved energy levels throughout the day. Remember to start with lighter weights and gradually increase weight as your strength improves to avoid injury.

Creating a Personalized Exercise Routine

CREATING a personalized exercise routine can be a great way to improve energy levels and overall health. Here are some steps to help you create a personalized exercise routine:

- Determine Your Goals: Before you start creating a workout routine, it's important to determine your goals. Are you looking to improve overall fitness, build strength, or increase endurance? Knowing your goals can help you choose the right exercises and develop a plan that is tailored to your needs.
- Assess Your Fitness Level: It's important to assess your current fitness level before starting any exercise program. This can include measurements like body weight, body fat percentage, and fitness tests like a timed run or a maximum lift. Knowing your starting point can help you track progress and adjust your routine as needed.
- Choose Your Exercises: Based on your goals and fitness level, choose exercises that are appropriate for your needs. This might include cardiovascular exercises like running or cycling, resistance training exercises like

weightlifting or bodyweight exercises, or flexibility exercises like yoga or stretching.

- Determine Frequency and Intensity: Determine how often you want to exercise and at what intensity. For example, you might aim for 30 minutes of moderate-intensity exercise five days a week, or 60 minutes of high-intensity exercise three days a week. It's important to choose a routine that is sustainable and achievable for you.

- Plan Your Workouts: Once you have chosen your exercises and determined your frequency and intensity, plan your workouts for the week. This might include specific exercises, sets, and reps, as well as warm-up and cool-down periods. Having a plan in place can help you stay on track and make progress towards your goals.

- Monitor Your Progress: Regularly monitor your progress to track your success and adjust your routine as needed. This might include tracking your workouts in a journal or app, taking measurements like body weight or body fat percentage, or performing fitness tests to see improvements in your strength or endurance.

Regular exercise is essential for maintaining optimal energy levels and overall health, so start today and enjoy the benefits of a healthy and active lifestyle.

Cold Therapy

Cold therapy, also known as cryotherapy, is a technique that involves exposing the body to cold temperatures to promote healing and reduce inflammation. While cold therapy is commonly used for pain relief and injury recovery, it can also be used to increase energy levels.

Cold therapy works by activating the body's natural healing response. When exposed to cold temperatures, the body responds by constricting blood vessels and reducing blood flow to the affected area. This reduces inflammation and promotes healing. The body also releases endorphins, which are natural painkillers that can promote feelings of wellbeing and increased energy levels.

There are several ways to incorporate cold therapy into your routine. One popular method is cold showers, which involves taking a shower with cold water for a period of time. This can be a quick and easy way to incorporate cold therapy into your daily routine. Another option is to use ice packs or cold compresses on specific areas of the body, such as the neck or face. This can be particularly effective for reducing headaches and promoting energy levels.

COLD THERAPY HAS BEEN SHOWN to have several benefits for energy levels. It can help to reduce fatigue and increase alertness, making it a great way to start the day. Cold therapy can also help to improve sleep quality, which can further improve energy levels.

WHILE COLD THERAPY can be an effective way to increase energy levels, it's important to use it safely. Always start with short exposure times and gradually increase the duration and intensity of your cold therapy sessions. It's also important to listen to your body and stop if you feel uncomfortable or experience any negative side effects.

COLD THERAPY IS a natural and effective way to increase energy levels. By activating the body's natural healing response and releasing endorphins, cold therapy can help to reduce inflammation, promote healing, and increase feelings of wellbeing and energy. Incorporating cold showers, ice packs, or other forms of cold therapy into your routine can help to improve energy levels and overall health.

If you want a deeper dive into cold therapy for stress reduction check out my companion book:

<u>The Cold Plunge Cryotherapy Book: Diving Into the Healing Powers of Cold Water Exposure</u>

by Hunter Hazelton

sleep and energy

. . .

"The measure of a man's real character is what he would do if he knew he would never be found out."

Thomas Babington Macaulay

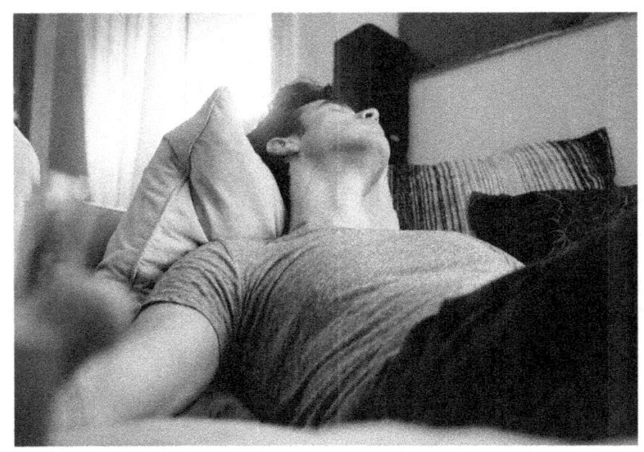

The Connection Between Sleep and Energy

SLEEP PLAYS a crucial role in our bodies' ability to produce and maintain energy levels. When we sleep, our bodies go through various stages of restorative processes that help to repair and replenish our cells and tissues. These processes are essential for energy production and overall health.

ONE IMPORTANT PROCESS that occurs during sleep is the release of growth hormone, which is essential for tissue repair and muscle growth. Growth hormone also helps to regulate metabolism, which is important for energy production. Without enough sleep, the release of growth hormone may be disrupted, leading to decreased energy levels and impaired recovery.

SLEEP ALSO HELPS to regulate the production of cortisol, a hormone that is released in response to stress. When cortisol levels are elevated for prolonged periods of time, it can lead to fatigue and decreased energy levels. Adequate sleep is essential for regulating cortisol levels and reducing stress, which can improve overall energy levels.

ANOTHER IMPORTANT ASPECT of sleep for energy production is the regulation of our circadian rhythms. Our circadian rhythms help to regulate our sleep-wake cycles, as well as many other physiological processes in the body. When our circadian rhythms are disrupted, it can lead to decreased energy levels and fatigue. By maintaining a regular sleep-wake schedule and getting enough sleep, we can help to regulate our circadian rhythms and improve energy levels.

IN ADDITION to the physiological processes that occur during sleep, our behaviors during the day can also impact our sleep quality and energy levels. For example, consuming caffeine or alcohol close to bedtime, engaging in stimulating activities like watching TV or using electronic devices, or exercising too close to bedtime can all disrupt sleep and lead to decreased energy levels the next day.

Tips for Better Sleep Quality

GETTING good quality sleep is essential for maintaining optimal energy levels and overall health. Here are some tips for improving sleep quality:

- Stick to a regular sleep schedule: Try to go to bed and wake up at the same time every day, even on weekends. This can help to regulate your body's internal clock and improve sleep quality.
- Create a relaxing bedtime routine: Develop a relaxing bedtime routine that helps you wind down before bed. This might include reading a book, taking a warm bath, or practicing relaxation techniques like meditation or deep breathing.
- Create a sleep-conducive environment: Make sure your bedroom is cool, dark, and quiet. Invest in comfortable bedding and pillows, and consider using blackout curtains or earplugs to block out noise and light.
- Avoid stimulating activities before bed: Avoid stimulating activities like watching TV, using electronic devices, or engaging in intense exercise before bed. These activities can interfere with sleep and make it harder to fall asleep.
- Limit caffeine and alcohol intake: Limit your intake of caffeine and alcohol, particularly in

the evening. These substances can interfere with sleep and lead to decreased energy levels the next day.

- Get regular exercise: Regular exercise can help to improve sleep quality, but it's important to avoid exercising too close to bedtime. Aim for moderate-intensity exercise during the day, and try to finish your workout at least a few hours before bedtime.

- Manage stress: Stress can interfere with sleep and lead to decreased energy levels. Practice stress management techniques like meditation, deep breathing, or yoga to help you relax and unwind before bed.

REMEMBER that good sleep habits take time to develop, so be patient and persistent in your efforts to improve your sleep quality. If you continue to struggle with sleep issues, consider talking to a healthcare provider for additional guidance and support.

Establishing a Sleep Routine for Maximum Energy

GETTING enough sleep is essential for maintaining maximum energy levels and overall health. However, it's not just about the quantity of sleep that we get, but also the quality. By establishing a consistent sleep routine, we can improve the quality of our sleep, which can lead to increased energy levels and improved overall health. In this article, we'll discuss some tips for establishing a sleep routine that can help you get the most out of your sleep.

Why is Sleep Important for Energy?

SLEEP IS important for many reasons, including cognitive functioning, immune function, and metabolism regulation. But, it's particularly important for energy production. During sleep, our bodies go through various restorative processes that help to repair and replenish our cells and tissues. This includes the release of growth hormone, which is essential for tissue repair and muscle growth. Growth hormone also helps to regulate metabolism, which is important for energy production. Adequate sleep is essential for regulating cortisol levels and reducing stress, which can improve overall energy levels. Without enough sleep, our bodies can't fully repair and replenish themselves, leading to decreased energy levels and impaired recovery.

Creating a Sleep-Conducive Environment

THE FIRST STEP in establishing a sleep routine is creating a sleep-conducive environment. A good sleep environment should be cool, dark, and quiet. It's important to invest in comfortable bedding and pillows to ensure maximum comfort. Consider using blackout curtains or eye masks to block out light, and earplugs or white noise machines to block out noise. A sleep-friendly environment can help to promote relaxation and reduce stress, making it easier to fall asleep and stay asleep.

Establishing a Sleep Schedule

ESTABLISHING a consistent sleep schedule is key to improving the quality of your sleep. Try to go to bed and wake up at the same time every day, even on weekends. This helps to regulate your body's internal clock and improve sleep quality. It's also important to create a relaxing bedtime routine that helps you wind down before bed. This might include reading a book, taking a warm bath, or practicing relaxation techniques like meditation or deep breathing.

Avoid Stimulating Activities Before Bed

AVOID STIMULATING activities like watching TV, using electronic devices, or engaging in intense exercise before bed. These activities can interfere with sleep and make it harder to fall asleep. Instead, focus on activities that promote relaxation, such as reading or taking a warm bath. It's also important to avoid consuming caffeine and alcohol, particularly in the evening. These substances can interfere with sleep and lead to decreased energy levels the next day.

Manage Stress

STRESS CAN INTERFERE with sleep and lead to decreased energy levels. It's important to develop strategies for managing stress, such as meditation, deep breathing, or yoga. These techniques can help to promote relaxation and reduce stress, making it easier to fall asleep and stay asleep. It's also important to avoid stressful activities before bed, such as work-related tasks or arguments with family members.

Regular Exercise

REGULAR EXERCISE CAN HELP to improve sleep quality, but it's important to avoid exercising too close to bedtime. Aim for moderate-intensity exercise during the day, and try to finish your workout at least a few hours before bedtime. Exercise can help to reduce stress and promote relaxation, making it easier to fall asleep and stay asleep.

The Importance of Consistency

CONSISTENCY IS key when it comes to establishing a sleep routine. It can take time for your body to adjust to a new sleep schedule, so it's important to be patient and persistent in your efforts. Stick to your sleep schedule as closely as possible, even on weekends. This will help to regulate your body's internal clock and improve sleep quality. If you do need to make changes to your sleep schedule, try to do so gradually, making small adjustments over time.

ESTABLISHING a consistent sleep routine is essential for maximum energy levels and overall health. Creating a sleep-conducive environment, establishing a sleep schedule, avoiding stimulating activities before bed, managing stress, and getting regular exercise are all important steps in developing a sleep routine that works for you. Remember that consistency is key, and it may take time for your body to adjust to a new sleep schedule. By making sleep a priority and taking steps to improve sleep quality, you can improve your energy levels and overall health. So, try these tips and see how they work for you, and be patient as you establish a sleep routine that works for you.

stress and energy

. . .

"A real man can't stand seeing his woman hurt. He's careful with his decisions and actions, so he never has to be responsible for her pain."

Denzel Washington

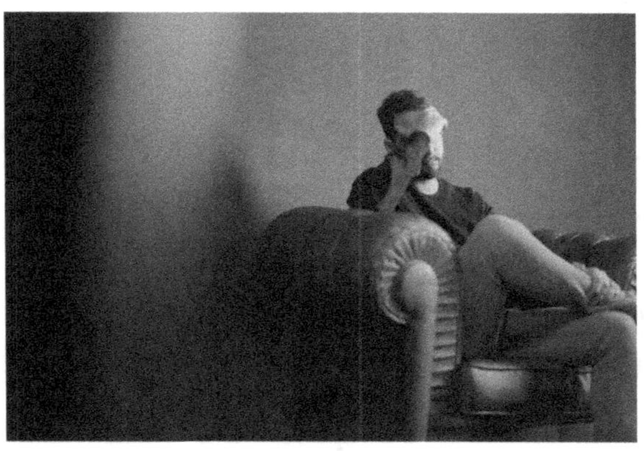

The Impact of Stress on Energy Levels

STRESS IS a normal part of life, and our bodies are equipped to handle small amounts of stress. However, chronic stress can have a significant impact on energy levels and overall health. When we experience stress, our bodies release hormones like cortisol and adrenaline, which can help us respond to the stressor. However, when stress is chronic, the constant release of these hormones can lead to fatigue and decreased energy levels.

CHRONIC STRESS CAN ALSO IMPACT sleep quality, which can further impact energy levels. When we're stressed, we may have trouble falling asleep or staying asleep, which can lead to daytime fatigue and decreased energy levels. Chronic stress can also interfere with the body's ability to repair and regenerate cells and tissues during sleep, which can further impact energy levels.

ANOTHER WAY that chronic stress can impact energy levels is by reducing our motivation and ability to engage in activities that promote energy, such as exercise or socializing. When we're stressed, we may feel overwhelmed and lack the motivation to engage in activities that we enjoy. This can lead to decreased energy levels and further exacerbate stress.

Chronic stress can also impact our diet, leading to poor food choices and decreased energy levels. When we're stressed, we may turn to comfort foods that are high in sugar and fat, which can lead to a temporary energy boost but ultimately lead to decreased energy levels. Chronic stress can also impact our appetite, leading to overeating or under-eating, which can further impact energy levels.

In addition to impacting energy levels, chronic stress can also have a negative impact on overall health. It can lead to a weakened immune system, increased inflammation, and an increased risk of chronic diseases like heart disease and diabetes.

Fortunately, there are steps we can take to reduce stress and improve energy levels. Some strategies for reducing stress include mindfulness meditation, deep breathing, and exercise. These activities can help to reduce stress and promote relaxation, leading to improved energy levels. It's also important to prioritize sleep and maintain a healthy diet, as these can also help to reduce stress and improve energy levels.

CHRONIC STRESS CAN HAVE a significant impact on energy levels and overall health. By recognizing the impact of stress on our bodies and taking steps to reduce stress, we can improve energy levels and overall health. Incorporating relaxation techniques, prioritizing sleep and a healthy diet, and engaging in regular exercise can all help to reduce stress and promote improved energy levels.

Techniques for Managing Stress

STRESS IS a common experience for many people, and it can have a significant impact on our energy levels, health, and overall wellbeing. While it may not be possible to completely eliminate stress from our lives, there are techniques that we can use to manage stress and reduce its impact on our lives. Here are some effective techniques for managing stress:

- Mindfulness meditation: Mindfulness meditation is a technique that involves focusing your attention on the present moment and accepting your thoughts and feelings without judgment. This can help to reduce stress and promote relaxation, leading to improved energy levels.

- Deep breathing: Deep breathing involves taking slow, deep breaths in through your nose and out through your mouth. This can help to reduce stress and promote relaxation, leading to improved energy levels.
- Exercise: Exercise is a powerful stress reducer, as it releases endorphins in the brain that promote feelings of happiness and wellbeing. Regular exercise can also improve sleep quality, which can further reduce stress and improve energy levels.
- Yoga: Yoga combines physical postures, breathing exercises, and meditation to promote relaxation and reduce stress. It can be an effective way to manage stress and improve energy levels.
- Social support: Spending time with friends and family can help to reduce stress and promote relaxation. Social support can also provide a sense of community and belonging, which can help to improve overall wellbeing and energy levels.
- Time management: Effective time management can help to reduce stress by reducing feelings of overwhelm and giving us

a sense of control over our lives. By prioritizing tasks and setting realistic goals, we can reduce stress and improve energy levels.

- Cognitive-behavioral therapy: Cognitive-behavioral therapy (CBT) is a form of therapy that focuses on changing negative thought patterns and behaviors that contribute to stress. It can be an effective way to manage stress and improve energy levels.

BY INCORPORATING these techniques into your daily routine, you can effectively manage stress and improve energy levels. It's important to remember that what works for one person may not work for another, so it may take some trial and error to find the techniques that work best for you. It's also important to prioritize self-care and make time for relaxation and stress reduction activities.

Mindfulness and Meditation Practices for Improved Energy and Focus

MINDFULNESS AND MEDITATION practices have become increasingly popular in recent years, and for good reason. These practices have been shown to improve focus, reduce stress, and increase overall energy levels. Here are some mindfulness and meditation practices that can help to improve energy and focus:

- Body scan meditation: Body scan meditation involves focusing your attention on different parts of your body, from your toes to the top of your head. This can help to increase awareness of your body and reduce stress, leading to improved energy levels.
- Breathing meditation: Breathing meditation involves focusing your attention on your breath and observing your thoughts as they come and go. This can help to reduce stress and improve focus, leading to improved energy levels.
- Walking meditation: Walking meditation involves walking slowly and mindfully, focusing your attention on each step and the sensations in your body. This can help to improve focus and reduce stress, leading to improved energy levels.
- Loving-kindness meditation: Loving-kindness meditation involves focusing your attention on feelings of love and kindness towards yourself and others. This can help to improve mood and reduce stress, leading to improved energy levels.

- Mindful eating: Mindful eating involves paying attention to the experience of eating, including the taste, texture, and smell of food. This can help to improve awareness of hunger and fullness cues, leading to improved energy levels.

INCORPORATING these practices into your daily routine can help to improve energy and focus. It's important to remember that mindfulness and meditation are skills that take practice, so be patient with yourself as you develop these practices. Start with short sessions and gradually increase the length of your practice as you become more comfortable. It's also important to make these practices a regular part of your routine to see the full benefits. By incorporating mindfulness and meditation practices into your daily routine, you can improve energy and focus and reduce stress.

If you want a deeper dive into mindfulness for stress reduction check out:

<u>Mindfulness Hacks for Men: Finding Peace and Presence in a Busy World</u>

by Harper Wells

hormones and energy

. . .

"The man who views the world at fifty the same as he did at twenty has wasted thirty years of his life."

Muhammad Ali

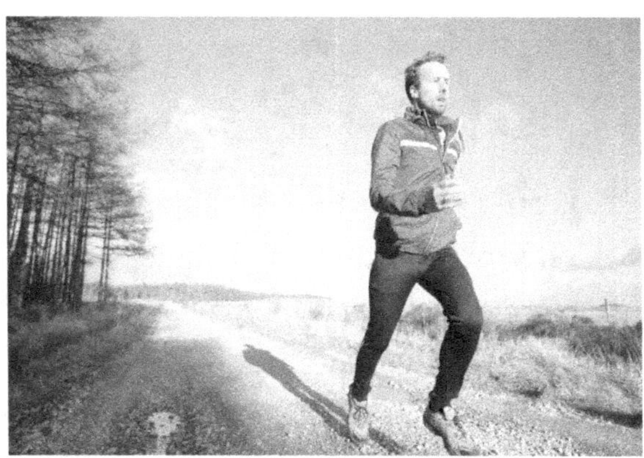

The Role of Hormones in Energy Levels

HORMONES ARE OFTEN FORGOTTEN when we think about low energy in men. These chemical messengers are produced by various glands in the endocrine system and help to regulate numerous bodily functions, including metabolism, growth and development, and stress response.

ONE OF THE most important hormones for energy levels is cortisol, which is produced by the adrenal glands. Cortisol plays a key role in the body's stress response, and helps to regulate blood sugar levels, blood pressure, and inflammation. However, chronic stress can lead to consistently high levels of cortisol, which can lead to fatigue and decreased energy levels.

ANOTHER IMPORTANT HORMONE for energy levels is insulin, which is produced by the pancreas. Insulin helps to regulate blood sugar levels by signaling cells to absorb glucose from the bloodstream. However, chronic insulin resistance, which is a common condition in people with type 2 diabetes, can lead to consistently high blood sugar levels and decreased energy levels.

TESTOSTERONE IS another hormone that plays a role in energy levels, particularly in men. Testosterone is produced by the testes and helps to regulate muscle mass, bone density, and sex drive. Low testosterone levels can lead to decreased energy levels, as well as other symptoms like decreased muscle mass and bone density.

ESTROGEN IS another hormone that plays a role in energy levels, particularly in women. Estrogen helps to regulate the menstrual cycle and promotes bone health. Low estrogen levels, particularly during menopause, can lead to decreased energy levels, as well as other symptoms like hot flashes and mood swings.

IN ADDITION TO THESE HORMONES, thyroid hormones also play a crucial role in regulating energy levels. The thyroid gland produces hormones that help to regulate metabolism, which is the process by which the body converts food into energy. Low thyroid hormone levels, a condition known as hypothyroidism, can lead to fatigue and decreased energy levels.

. . .

IN CONCLUSION, hormones play a crucial role in regulating energy levels in the body. Cortisol, insulin, testosterone, estrogen, and thyroid hormones all play a role in regulating metabolism, blood sugar levels, and other bodily functions that impact energy levels. By maintaining hormone balance through healthy lifestyle habits like exercise, stress management, and a balanced diet, we can promote optimal energy levels and overall health.

Identifying Hormonal Imbalances that Cause Low Energy

IDENTIFYING hormonal imbalances that cause low energy can be challenging, as many of the symptoms of hormonal imbalances can be vague and difficult to pinpoint. However, there are some practical tips that can help you to notice low energy and potential hormonal imbalances:

- Keep a journal: Keeping a journal of your symptoms can help you to identify patterns and potential triggers for low energy. Note when you feel most fatigued, what you ate, how much sleep you got, and any other relevant factors.

- Get tested: If you suspect that you may have a hormonal imbalance, talk to your healthcare provider about getting tested. Blood tests can help to identify imbalances in hormones like cortisol, insulin, testosterone, estrogen, and thyroid hormones.

- Notice changes in energy levels: Pay attention to changes in your energy levels throughout the day. If you notice that you consistently feel tired in the afternoon or have trouble falling asleep at night, this could be a sign of a hormonal imbalance.

- Monitor your diet: A healthy diet is crucial for hormone balance, so pay attention to what you're eating. Eating too much sugar or refined carbohydrates can lead to blood sugar imbalances and decreased energy levels.

- Evaluate your sleep habits: Poor sleep quality can impact hormone balance and energy levels. Evaluate your sleep habits and make changes if necessary, such as creating a sleep-conducive environment or establishing a regular sleep routine.

- Manage stress: Chronic stress can impact hormone balance and energy levels. Identify sources of stress in your life and take steps to manage them, such as practicing relaxation techniques or engaging in regular exercise.

By PAYING attention to changes in your energy levels, monitoring your diet and sleep habits, and managing stress, you can help to identify potential hormonal imbalances that may be contributing to low energy. If you suspect that you have a hormonal imbalance, talk to your healthcare provider about getting tested and developing a plan to restore hormone balance and improve energy levels.

Strategies for Balancing Hormones Naturally

BALANCING hormones naturally can help to improve energy levels, mood, and overall wellbeing. You will notice that many of the strategies to balancing hormones naturally are the same strategies that deal with our overall energy levels previously discussed. Think of this as the giant blinking sign in the book to remind you that our bodies work as a machine and all aspects must be in sync for optimal balance and health.

· · ·

ONE OF THE most important strategies for balancing hormones naturally is to eat a balanced diet. This means consuming plenty of whole foods, healthy fats, and lean proteins, while avoiding processed foods and excess sugar. A diet that is rich in nutrients can help to support hormone balance and reduce inflammation.

ANOTHER IMPORTANT STRATEGY for balancing hormones naturally is to manage stress. Chronic stress can disrupt hormone balance, so it's important to find ways to manage stress. Techniques like meditation, yoga, and deep breathing can be effective for reducing stress and promoting relaxation.

REGULAR EXERCISE IS another important strategy for balancing hormones naturally. Exercise helps to reduce stress, promote relaxation, and regulate blood sugar levels, all of which can help to support hormone balance. Aim for at least 30 minutes of moderate exercise most days of the week.

SLEEP IS ALSO crucial for hormone balance. Aim for 7-9 hours of sleep per night and establish a regular sleep routine to support healthy sleep patterns.

. . .

FINALLY, natural supplements and herbs can also help to support hormone balance. These include supplements like omega-3 fatty acids, vitamin D, and magnesium, as well as herbs like ashwagandha and maca root.

IT's important to remember that hormone balance is a complex process, and there is no one-size-fits-all approach. It's always a good idea to work with a health-care provider who can help to identify any hormonal imbalances and develop a personalized plan to restore hormone balance and improve overall health and wellbeing.

lifestyle changes for more energy

· · ·

"Real men don't dance to other people's tune, instead they create their own rhythm and others follow."

Gift Gugu Mona

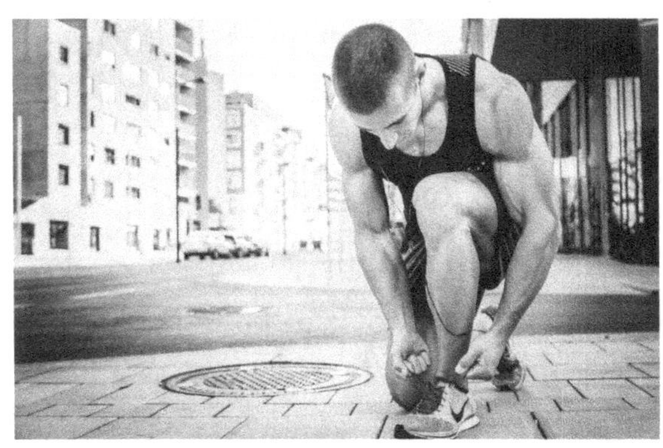

Making Sustainable Lifestyle Changes for Increased Energy

MAKING sustainable lifestyle changes for increased energy can be challenging, but it's important to focus on specific strategies that can be maintained over time. Here are some specific strategies men can utilize for making sustainable lifestyle changes for increased energy:

- Establish a regular sleep routine: Establishing a regular sleep routine is crucial for improving energy levels. Go to bed and wake up at the same time each day, even on weekends, to establish a consistent sleep-wake cycle. Create a sleep-conducive environment by keeping your bedroom cool, dark, and quiet, and avoid screens and stimulating activities before bed.
- Incorporate movement into your day: Regular physical activity is important for improving energy levels. Find activities that you enjoy, such as jogging, cycling, or weight lifting, and incorporate them into your daily routine. Take breaks throughout the day to

stretch or go for a walk, and consider incorporating physical activity into your daily routine, such as cycling or walking to work.

- Stay hydrated: Dehydration can lead to fatigue and decreased energy levels. Aim for at least 8 glasses of water per day, and carry a water bottle with you to stay hydrated on-the-go. Avoid sugary drinks and excessive alcohol, which can lead to dehydration.

- Eat a balanced diet: A balanced diet is crucial for improving energy levels. Focus on whole, nutrient-dense foods like fruits, vegetables, whole grains, lean proteins, and healthy fats. Avoid processed foods and excessive sugar, which can disrupt hormone balance and lead to inflammation.

- Manage stress: Chronic stress can lead to fatigue and decreased energy levels. Incorporate stress-reducing activities into your routine, such as meditation, yoga, or deep breathing exercises. Take breaks throughout the day to relax and engage in activities that you enjoy.

- Build a support system: Building a support system can help you to stay accountable and motivated. Surround yourself with friends and family who support your goals and encourage you to make positive changes.

Consider joining a support group or working with a coach to help you stay on track.

REMEMBER to be patient with yourself and celebrate small successes along the way. Over time, these small changes can add up to significant improvements in energy levels and overall health and wellbeing.

Managing Energy Levels at Work

IT'S A BUSY WORKDAY, and you're feeling the drag of low energy. You've got deadlines looming, meetings to attend, and your coffee cup is empty. But fear not, my friends, for I have some tips to help you manage your energy levels and conquer the day like a boss.

FIRST THINGS FIRST, let's talk about sleep. We all know that a good night's sleep is crucial for energy, but how do you get it? Well, let me tell you, it's all about routine. Establish a regular sleep routine and create a sleep-conducive environment. Turn off the screens, darken the room, and put on some soothing music. You'll be sleeping like a baby in no time.

. . .

Now, onto breakfast. They say it's the most important meal of the day, and for good reason. A balanced breakfast sets you up for success by giving you the energy you need to power through your day. So ditch the sugary cereals and opt for something with protein, healthy fats, and whole grains. Your body will thank you.

BUT WHAT ABOUT when you hit that mid-morning slump? Fear not, my friends, for I have a solution. It's called the power nap. Find a quiet place, close your eyes, and let yourself drift off for 20-30 minutes. When you wake up, you'll feel refreshed and ready to tackle the rest of your day.

Now, let's talk about hydration. Dehydration can lead to fatigue, so make sure to drink plenty of water throughout the day. Keep a water bottle on hand and take frequent sips. And if you're feeling really adventurous, try adding some lemon or cucumber slices for a refreshing twist.

BUT WHAT ABOUT when the day starts to drag on? That's when it's time to get moving. Take a break and stretch your legs, or better yet, do some jumping jacks or push-ups. It might sound silly, but trust me, it works. Getting your blood flowing will help you feel more alert and energized.

AND LAST BUT NOT LEAST, let's talk about mindset. The way you think about your day can have a big impact on your energy levels. If you're feeling overwhelmed, take a deep breath and remind yourself that you can do this. Focus on one task at a time and celebrate small victories along the way. You'll be amazed at how much of a difference a positive attitude can make.

SO THERE YOU HAVE IT, my friends. Some simple tips to help you manage your energy levels and conquer your busy workday. Remember, it's all about routine, hydration, movement, and mindset. So go forth, be productive, and kick some butt. You've got this.

Incorporating Fun and Relaxation into Your Life

INCORPORATING fun and relaxation into your life is crucial for maintaining a healthy work-life balance and managing stress. It can be easy to get caught up in the daily grind of work and responsibilities, but taking time for yourself to unwind and have fun can actually help you be more productive in the long run. Here are some tips for incorporating fun and relaxation into your life:

- Schedule it in: Just like you would schedule a meeting or appointment, schedule in time for fun and relaxation. This could be anything from taking a yoga class to going to a movie or spending time with friends. Make it a priority and don't let work or other obligations get in the way.
- Find activities you enjoy: Think about activities that bring you joy and make you feel relaxed. This could be anything from reading a book to going for a hike or trying a new hobby. Find what works for you and make it a regular part of your routine.
- Unplug: In our constantly connected world, it can be hard to unplug and disconnect. But taking a break from technology can be incredibly refreshing and relaxing. Try setting aside some time each day to disconnect from your phone, computer, and other devices.
- Get outside: Spending time in nature can be incredibly restorative and relaxing. Whether it's going for a walk in the park or taking a camping trip, getting outside can help you recharge and feel more energized.

- Laugh: Laughter is the best medicine, as they say. Find ways to inject humor and laughter into your day, whether it's watching a funny movie or telling jokes with friends.
- Practice mindfulness: Mindfulness practices like meditation or deep breathing can help you relax and reduce stress. Try incorporating mindfulness into your daily routine, even if it's just a few minutes each day.

INCORPORATING fun and relaxation into your life doesn't have to be complicated or time-consuming. By scheduling in time for yourself, finding activities you enjoy, unplugging, getting outside, laughing, and practicing mindfulness, you can improve your overall well-being and manage stress more effectively.

maintaining your energy long-term

. . .

"The strength of a man isn't seen in the power of his arms. It's seen in the love with which he embraces you."

Steve Maraboli

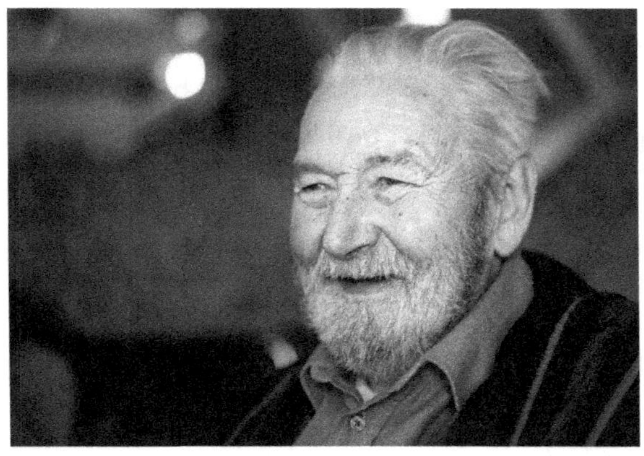

How to Prioritize Energy and Maintain Healthy Habits

LISTEN UP, my friends. It's time to prioritize your energy and maintain healthy habits like a boss. But how, you ask? Fear not, for I have some tips to help you do just that.

FIRST THINGS FIRST, let's talk about sleep. You can't prioritize your energy if you're not getting enough shut-eye. Establish a regular sleep routine and create a sleep-conducive environment. Get cozy, turn off those screens, and let yourself drift off into dreamland.

BUT WHAT ABOUT when you wake up feeling groggy and sluggish? Fear not, my friends, for I have a solution. It's called breakfast. That's right, the most important meal of the day. Make sure to fuel up with a balanced breakfast that includes protein, healthy fats, and whole grains. Your body will thank you.

. . .

Now, let's talk about movement. Regular physical activity is crucial for maintaining energy levels and overall health. Find activities that you enjoy, like lifting weights or going for a run, and make them a regular part of your routine. And don't forget to take breaks throughout the day to stretch or go for a quick walk. Your body will thank you.

But what about when you're feeling overwhelmed with work and responsibilities? It's time to prioritize your time, my friends. Make a list of your priorities and schedule them in. Focus on the most important tasks first and don't let distractions get in the way. And don't forget to take breaks throughout the day to recharge and refocus.

Now, let's talk about nutrition. Eating a balanced diet is crucial for maintaining energy levels and overall health. Focus on whole, nutrient-dense foods like fruits, vegetables, lean proteins, and healthy fats. And don't forget to stay hydrated by drinking plenty of water throughout the day.

But what about when you're feeling stressed and overwhelmed? It's time to take a break, my friends. Incorporate relaxation and stress-reducing activities into your routine, like yoga, meditation, or deep breathing exercises. Take time for yourself to unwind and recharge.

. . .

AND LAST BUT NOT LEAST, let's talk about mindset. The way you think about your energy and habits can have a big impact on your success. Believe in yourself and your ability to prioritize your energy and maintain healthy habits. Celebrate small successes along the way and stay motivated by visualizing your goals.

SO THERE YOU HAVE IT. Some simple tips to help you prioritize your energy and maintain healthy habits like a boss. Remember, it's all about sleep, breakfast, movement, time management, nutrition, relaxation, and mindset. You've got this.

Benefits of Sustained High Energy Levels

SUSTAINED high energy levels can have a significant impact on a man's overall health and well-being. Here are just a few of the benefits:

- Increased productivity: High energy levels can increase a man's productivity, allowing him to get more done in less time. This can lead to greater success at work and in other areas of life.

- Improved physical performance: When a man has high energy levels, he is more likely to perform better physically, whether during exercise or everyday activities. He'll have more stamina and endurance, allowing him to push himself further and accomplish more.
- Better mood: Low energy levels can contribute to feelings of fatigue, irritability, and even depression. On the other hand, sustained high energy levels can improve a man's mood and overall sense of well-being.
- Improved cognitive function: When a man has high energy levels, he is able to think more clearly and make better decisions. This can lead to improved cognitive function and better problem-solving skills.
- Better sleep: Sustained high energy levels can also improve a man's sleep quality. When he has more energy during the day, he'll be more likely to feel tired and ready for bed at night, leading to better sleep and overall restfulness.
- Increased confidence: When a man feels energized and capable, he is more likely to have confidence in himself and his abilities. This can lead to greater success and fulfillment in all areas of life.

- Improved relationships: When a man has high energy levels, he is more likely to be engaged and present in his relationships with others. This can lead to improved communication, better connections, and stronger relationships overall.

IN SUMMARY, sustained high energy levels can improve a man's productivity, physical performance, mood, cognitive function, sleep quality, confidence, and relationships.

Tracking Progress and Staying Motivated

TRACKING your progress and staying motivated is crucial for maintaining high energy levels and making sustainable lifestyle changes. Here are a few strategies for doing just that:

- Set specific goals: Identify specific, measurable goals that you want to achieve, whether it's losing weight, increasing your strength, or improving your sleep habits.

Write them down and track your progress over time.

- Use a tracking system: Use a tracking system to monitor your progress towards your goals. This could be a journal, an app, or a spreadsheet. Update it regularly and review your progress regularly to stay motivated.
- Celebrate small victories: Celebrate your small victories along the way. Every time you hit a milestone or achieve a small goal, take a moment to acknowledge and celebrate it. This can help keep you motivated and on track.
- Find a support system: Surround yourself with people who support your goals and encourage you to stay on track. This could be a workout partner, a friend or family member, or an online community. Having a support system can make a big difference in staying motivated and accountable.
- Mix things up: Keep things interesting by mixing up your routine and trying new things. This could be a new workout routine, a new healthy recipe, or a new relaxation technique. Variety can help keep you motivated and prevent boredom.
- Visualize success: Visualize yourself achieving your goals and living a healthy, energetic life.

> This can help keep you motivated and
> focused on your goals.

BY SETTING SPECIFIC GOALS, tracking your progress, celebrating small victories, finding a support system, mixing things up, and visualizing success, you can stay motivated and on track towards sustained high energy levels and overall health and well-being.

ANOTHER STRATEGY for tracking progress and staying motivated is to focus on the benefits of your efforts. For example, if you're working on improving your nutrition, focus on how much better you feel when you eat healthy foods, or how much more energy you have throughout the day. By focusing on the positive outcomes of your efforts, you can stay motivated to continue making healthy choices.

ANOTHER STRATEGY IS to reward yourself for your progress. Set up a system where you reward yourself for reaching certain milestones. For example, if you stick to your workout routine for a month, treat yourself to a massage or a new piece of workout gear. This can help keep you motivated and provide a tangible incentive to continue working towards your goals.

. . .

ADDITIONALLY, it's important to stay flexible and adjust your goals as needed. If you find that a particular strategy isn't working for you, don't be afraid to pivot and try something new. The key is to stay committed to your overall goal of sustained high energy levels and overall health and well-being.

FINALLY, don't forget to practice self-compassion. Making lifestyle changes can be challenging, and setbacks are a normal part of the process. When you experience setbacks, don't beat yourself up. Instead, focus on what you can learn from the experience and use it as motivation to continue moving forward.

IN SUMMARY, tracking progress and staying motivated are key strategies for maintaining sustained high energy levels and making healthy lifestyle changes. By setting specific goals, using a tracking system, celebrating small victories, finding a support system, visualizing success, focusing on the benefits of your efforts, rewarding yourself, staying flexible, and practicing self-compassion, you can stay motivated and on track towards a healthier, more energetic life.

conclusion

. . .

"The greatness of a man is not in how much wealth he acquires, but in his integrity and his ability to affect those around him positively."

Bob Marley

IN CONCLUSION, we have discussed a variety of key concepts and strategies for boosting energy levels and maintaining sustained high energy throughout our lives. From the importance of energy for men's health and well-being to the science behind energy production, and from the role of nutrition and exercise in energy production to the impact of stress and hormones on energy levels, we have explored a range of factors that can affect our energy levels and how we can take steps to improve them.

We have discussed the benefits of sustained high energy levels, including increased productivity, better mood, improved physical performance, and stronger relationships. We have also explored specific strategies for making sustainable lifestyle changes, such as setting specific goals, using a tracking system, celebrating small victories, finding a support system, mixing things up, and visualizing success.

Ultimately, the key takeaway is the importance of prioritizing our energy levels for a happier, healthier life. By making conscious choices about our nutrition, exercise, sleep, stress management, and other factors that affect our energy levels, we can improve our overall well-being and achieve greater success and fulfillment in all areas of life.

So, let's prioritize our energy levels and make sustainable lifestyle changes that will help us achieve our goals and live our best lives. Whether it's through exercise, nutrition, mindfulness practices, or other strategies, let's take the necessary steps to boost our energy levels and maintain sustained high energy for a happier, healthier life.

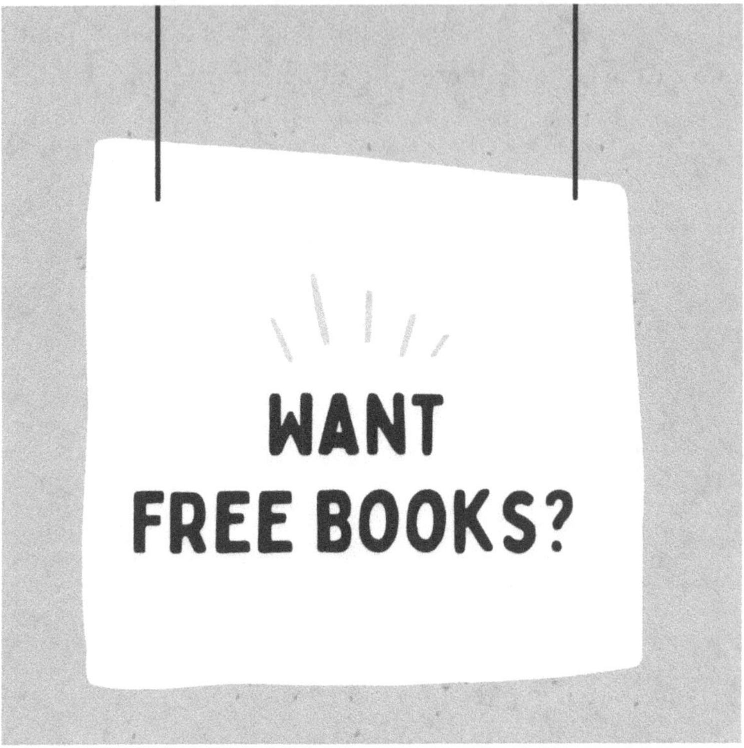

WANT
FREE BOOKS?
FREEBOOKDAILY.COM